MORE PRE
1949
ACUPUNCTURE

MORE PRE 1949 ACUPUNCTURE

Andrew McPherson

CONTENTS

PREFACE

After publishing my previous book, *Pre 1949 Acupuncture*, I have received a lot of enquiries regarding the subject. Hence, I am once again putting pen to paper to look at the issue in greater depth. If the reader is still unclear, I can only say that this is not only a difficult subject to teach but is also to discuss. This does not mean the topic of pre 1949 acupuncture is lacking in importance, just that there are many times in Chinese language which fail to have an adequate English language counterpart.

Since the task of writing about pre 1949 acupuncture has been left up to me, so it has been up to my wife and students, especially Anne Chalmers, to take on the enormous job of directly and indirectly helping in the production of this book. Many thanks.

Andrew McPherson

INTRODUCTION

By now, many readers, especially if they've read my last book, *Pre 1949 Acupuncture*, will have realised that acupuncture is more than just "sticking pins in people" and more than just fixing knees and fixing backs. It really depends on whether you "hold yourself up" as a doctor of Chinese medicine or simply an acupuncture therapist as most people really are today.

When discussing pre 1949 acupuncture with my patients who were medical researchers and PhD (in medical laboratory science) students and seeing what their responses were to the idea of treating people according to the time of day, etc., they were unanimous. They felt if this was the case, in fact, the reason must be "biorhythms"!

What made this answer so amazing was threefold. Firstly, I knew that research at an Australian university (unnamed) has recently found while bacteria didn't have "individual" consciousnesses (of course not), they did have "group" consciousnesses and are able to "get away" from the effects of "oncoming" antibiotics. Secondly, I came across a news report, not long ago, from a university in Chicago that bacteria were significantly influenced by "biorhythms". As if these weren't "enough", by themselves, it has also been reported on Australian government TV (i.e., The ABC) that research has shown that when children are born, they are not only covered in blood, amniotic fluid, and their mother's faces but, as a result, were covered from head-to-toe in bacteria. In actuality, the bacteria are two to three times the number of body cells of the newborn. Furthermore, according to scientific research, these bacteria have a profound effect on the baby's further development and what diseases it will get or not get in future. Does this not correspond to the Chinese views on birth previously classified as "superstitious"? (see Figure 1)

Figure 1

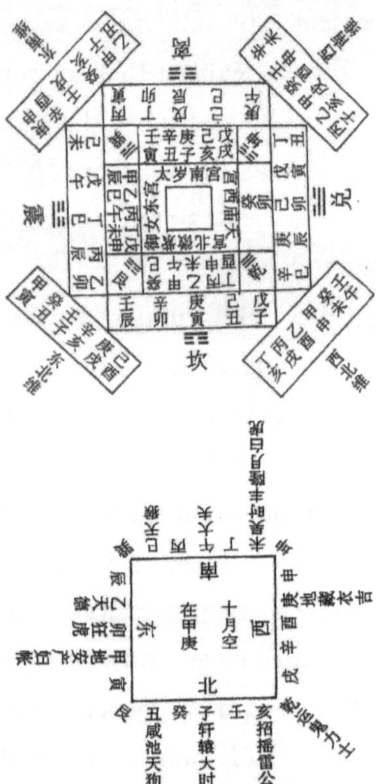

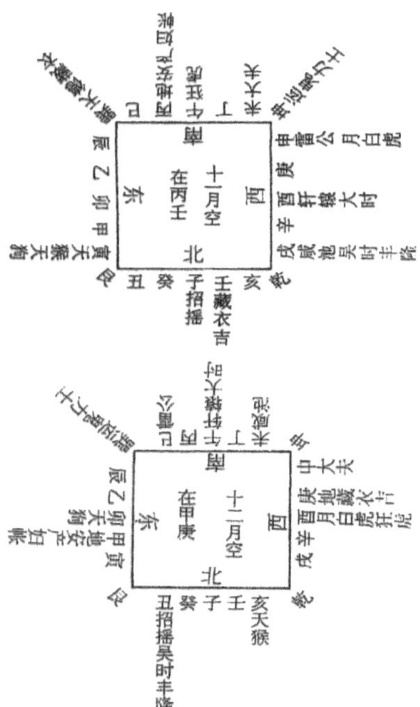

Insofar as this connection between nature and acupuncture, these are not the only examples that can be found. "Directions" play a big part in both pre 1949 acupuncture as well as in nature. Just as many programmes on TV show us that cows, left alone in fields will, as a matter of intuition, face north (unless there are overhead power lines) and dogs will squat to go the toilet again facing north (unless there is a lot of solar eruptions at the time), truly traditional acupuncture is also concerned with directions that represent that particular year and the different winds that come from various directions that affect each and every *iie qi* (the 24 climatic periods).

While on the subject of "winds", it is of even greater interest that the winds that blow in Greece were considered "evil" winds, but really, the authorities during WW1 were simply concerned with burying the bodies of fallen soldiers before the fleas on rats could be carried by the winds and spread septicaemic plague. Maybe those old wives' tales weren't so wrong after all.

In conclusion, acupuncture, as a system of treatment, is, of course, very advanced anyway. While Western medicine has been offering overly simplistic explanations for the successes of acupuncture since its big "discovery" in the 1970s, increasing evidence has "come forward," challenging these views. For example, significant university research in the United States, from an early stage, showed that the "neural-gate" theory and "endorphins" etc. didn't work the way we were told. Further research by the Chinese in the late 1970s also showed this. In other words, if you induce pain, from needles, it doesn't make you less sensitive and reduce overall pain conditions. In fact, it makes you more sensitive!

Coupled with this, there are studies done in Versailles, France, where small harmless radioactive particles have been injected into humans. It was found that these particles, when injected into areas where the Chinese don't mention channel activity, just remain inert. When they were injected into "channels", they flowed around the body accordingly. In addition, they flowed faster and faster on the fluoroscopes etc. when needled.

Now that we find ourselves more "entrenched" in the workings of 22nd-century life, we are using acupuncture and Chinese herbal medicine for the treatment of diseases, such as infertility. What does this have to do with the "neural-gate" or "endorphins" and the treatment of pain? Doesn't it beg to differ on the way or ways acupuncture really works? One never knows what acupuncture and Chinese herbs may be able to cure next.

CHAPTER 1

The Cause of Anger is The Liver and the Cause of Worry is The Lungs?

I could "go on" about how Western medicine is only just beginning to see that Chinese medicine is correct regarding the function of the spleen. Hitherto, the spleen was considered simply to be an outdated appendage from a bygone era. Only recently has Western medicine begun to appreciate it and realises that spleen is quite important (as is the case in traditional Chinese medicine) and is responsible for one's immunity and the production of B-cells (a marker used in HIV and AIDS).

I could also point out that acupuncture and, more precisely, Chinese herbs are not given proper credit when it comes to the treatment of cancer, tumours, and Parkinson's disease. How has the research into the use of snakes, scorpions, spiders, etc. (used in traditional Chinese medicine for 5,000 years), for a long time, been heralded as a great advance in Western science?

However, the object of this book is not to point out acupuncture's or Chinese herbal medicine's benefits (which are many) or to point out Western medicine's shortcomings (which are many). Rather, it is to emphasise and further explain the differences between acupuncture, which is widely taught today in colleges throughout the world, and pre 1949 acupuncture.

While it is quite difficult to describe pre 1949 acupuncture, as I've said previously, it is easier to tell the reader what it's not. Such is the case with emotions like "anger," "worry," etc. Take "anger" to begin with.

Any discussion, even about emotions, does, of course, require, firstly and foremost, a definition of the subject. In ancient times, there is surprisingly little said about "anger," and most references to the emotion are made to "xin fan" or "fan xin" (upset or irritable). Over the centuries, various other references have been made to "anger": "yi nu", "shan nu" (both meaning "easily angry"), "fan zao" (impatient), "fen fen" (like "nu"), "zao rao" (rashness or rage), etc.

Of course, there is one actual reference to "anger", as such, in the classics. As stated, "excess" syndromes of the liver can result in "anger" (just like "deficiency" syndromes can cause "fear").

There is also the implication that true "anger" involves shouting. Whether this is correct or not, there is no doubt that anger can be attributed to a lot of organ and channel dysfunctions. For example, the *Qian jin fang* (Sun Si miao) clearly states that "anger" can be a symptom of heart deficiency cold, small intestines yang illness, spleen muscle ji (weakness), lung excess heat, lung deficiency cold, zhi qi (accumulation), kidney jing problems, kidney excess heat, kidney lao (wasting) heat, etc.

In addition to "anger", we could just as easily look at "worry". Chinese medicine students normally associate "worry" with the lungs. However, rather than simply aiming at some sort of "knee-jerk" reaction to "worry" and, thereby, assuming there must be a lung problem, we perhaps should look a bit further. Again, as well as questioning what "worry" is in the first place, the *Qian jin fang* additionally reports that "worry" can be a symptom of gall bladder marrow deficiency, heart deficiency cold, small intestines wind dian, spleen deficient cool, kidney deficiency cool, etc.

Well then, if "anger" and "worry" are not always associated with the liver or the lungs respectively, what then? To understand this, we really need to go back to the early writings of acupuncture and Chinese medicine. It is only in the proper context can we understand these things.

The original Chinese writings regarding these emotions refer to the soul (hun) being housed in the liver; the spirit (shen), the heart; the ideas (yi), the spleen; the animal spirit (po), the lungs; and the will/purpose (zhi), the kidneys.

The original writings (in fact, part of the discussions between Qi bo and the Yellow Emperor in the *Su wen*) also talk about the Zang (organs) shapes showing not only in the body pulses but in the radial pulses as well. In reality, it records the use of cun, guan, chi (inch, bar, cubit) and the three parts: floating, middle, and sunken (fou, zhong, chen), thereby totalling nine hou. Although this idea is more fully enumerated in the *Xue gu zhen ci*, it is also described, in a similar vein, in the *Su wen* and later in the *Zhen jiu jia yi jing* (by Huang Fu mi).

Yes, I know I said in my previous book, *Pre 1949 Acupuncture*, doctors in the past didn't use the radial pulse as much as they used the body pulses, but wait one minute! While these "spirits" or emotions are housed in the organs, there is nothing to stop these spirits, etc., from "coming out" of these organs if induced to do so by diet, extreme weather, and by allowing oneself to be affected by emotional upheaval:

Table 1

RADIAL PULSES RE QI BO

	CUN	GUAN	CHI
TIAN (FLOATING)	HEAD CORNERS (GB)	LUNGS	LIVER
DI (MIDDLE)	MOUTH, TEETH (ST)	CHEST QI	KIDNEYS
REN (SUNKEN)	EARS, EYES (TH)	HEART	SPLEEN & STOMACH

Not only can these "spirits"/emotions etc. become "extreme", but like "bubbles", they can burst according to the time of the year and from year to year. (In traditional times, the Chinese and Japanese people, on the contrary, disliked emotional outbursts and instead tried to "maintain face".) Let's consider then the patient who is very "willful" when young, but he/she has little or no will when older. Why, therefore, do not all the radial pulses reflect the "truth" when taken? This is because the experienced doctor of acupuncture or Chinese medicine has to negotiate his/her way through a veritable minefield of radial pulses that are forceful or weak in keeping with, as I've said, the time of the year and year to year and avoiding distractions like "ni" (adversity, inverse conditions – deficiency or otherwise), "wang" (flare-ups), etc.

In other words, the acupuncturist should listen to the patient carefully and use maybe many, many means at his/her disposal to ascertain what's happened and why. Therefore, the idea that "anger" reflects the condition of the liver and "worry" reflects the condition of the lungs is pretty simplistic at best.

On the one hand, if the patient presents with a dry, hacking cough or, alternatively, a productive phlegmatic cough and is "worried", yes,

I might think this is from the lungs, particularly, if it's the time of the year with a lot of lung problems or, say, Autumn. On the other hand, if the "worry" is accompanied by other symptoms, pulses, etc., I might not be convinced to support the "lung" hypothesis.

Obviously, the modern Chinese, to simplify things, just "watered down" the classics and perhaps "too basically" taught people that "anger" related to the liver and "worry" related to the lungs.

CHAPTER 2

ST36 Is for Energy?

ST36 point (zu san li), is it for giving a patient energy? This would seem a rather rhetorical question. Every student of acupuncture, from an early stage in his/her studies, knows that this is the case. Or is it?

It is true that ST36 is good for many things. As the Chinese encyclopaedias on the subject list, ST36 can treat "abdomen inside cold, distended stuffy, borborygmus, abdomen pain, chest abdomen inside stagnant blood, smaller abdomen distended, skin swelling yin qi not enough, smaller abdomen hard, hot illness sweating can't reduce, easily vomiting, mouth bitter, body adverse injured, mouth shut, waist pain can't bend, easily sad/unhappy, breast swelling, throat bi and can't talk, stomach qi not enough, long-time dysentery, food can't transform, below ribs stuffy, knees cold atrophy, heat inside digests 'grains' poorly, abdomen hot, body upset, crazy talking, breast carbuncle, tendency to burp, dislikes food smells, crazy singing delusions and laughing/smiling, fear and anger and big complaining/abusing, cholera, bed-wetting, loss of qi, yang jue, afraid of cold, dizziness, urine can't unblock, etc." In addition, ST36 is often cited for the treatment of long-term chronic diseases and for removing "deficiency and excess evils".

After all this, one would think that ST36 is good for treating just about everything. However, this is not the case. For example, to mention a case in point, a patient seeking treatment from the author complained frequently about mainly feeling tired. After being treated a number of times with ST36, she failed to improve or not much. Upon further examination, it was found that the patient had a strong or almost forceful pulse (not as weak or deficient as expected) and a greasy tongue, especially at the back (not pale also as expected). Finally, the patient revealed she had had (until recently) cervical cancer. Suddenly, this all made a lot of sense: Her tiredness was due to cancer or its after-effects. ST36, on the other hand, is not really for this type of condition or this type of problem. Treating the affected area or using anti-cancer herbs, or better still considering the many imbalances that contributed to the problem in the first place, would have been more help. In addition, there is a lot of modern Western research that shows people who have cancer get anaemia and that Western doctors don't really know why. Some think it is from minute but continuous bleeding internally.

Either way, ST36 is mainly effective because it is the he-sea point (or ru point, i.e., the "enter" point) on the stomach channel. It also connects, by way of collaterals, to the spleen and kidney channels (see *On the Theory and Clinical Application of Channels and Collaterals* by Professor Guan Zun hui). These things do not mean that it can treat this problem. If the patient has poor absorption of or not enough food (as was commonly the case in ancient China) or is even constitutionally weak (as the Chinese doctors say is the situation with weak "kidneys"), then ST36 might help (and usually does).

Hence, in conclusion, we can see that ST36 is not a cure-all for all people and all diseases. Instead, we need to treat people according to their real conditions and not rely on point "indications". In other words, the point is not going to cure people; you, as a practitioner, are.

CHAPTER 3

Baldness Is Caused by Kidney Deficiency

By "kidney deficiency", we are talking about, from a Chinese point of view, the functions of the adrenal glands, the sexual organs (the gonads), the bones, the brain, and the kidneys themselves. However, we would be wrong assuming all baldness is from the "kidneys".

Yes, certainly, the classics (e.g., the *Neijing*) talk about baldness and hair loss in women being due to a problem with the "kidneys". And clinically, I confirm this. Many women came to my Chinese herbal medicine teacher, Dr. Kwai Lin lau, and myself over the years for hair loss, etc. (I can happily report that all recovered.) When women approach menopause (i.e., 40 years old or more), their oestrogen levels drop down, thereby increasing their male hormones by default. This directly or indirectly relates to the "kidneys", whether it is ultimately due to blood heat, blood loss, infection, etc. (all of which can affect the "blood" level and affect the "kidneys").

As far as men are concerned (and remember that it is of interest to the author being somewhat "follicularly-challenged"), it is another matter. Western medicine concludes hair loss is due not to too much sebum, as originally believed, but rather due to an allergic reaction to one's own sebum; so much so that instead of referring to alopecia as *alopecia seborrhoeica* (which was the case at the turn of the 20th century), it now refers to the problem as *alopecia androgenetica* (refer to *Recent Advances in Dermatology 4*).

In other words, instead of being considered a disease by Western medicine, it is more viewed as an immunity defect or as a result of racial type (not unlike some breeds of cat).

Chinese medicine, in fact, states in the classics that there are many causes of this "condition". Some books like the *Zhu bing yuan hou lun* believe that hair loss is due to heart lao (exhaustion and wasting). On the other hand, the *Qian jin fang* considers this to be a symptom of (heart mai ji).

Ultimately, whatever Western medicine or more modern (post 1949) Chinese medicine thinks regarding hair loss is not really the point. As Professor Guan Zun hui said to me in a lecture about the subject in 1989, true Chinese medicine and acupuncture (i.e., pre 1949 Acupuncture) is very different from Western medicine. While Western medicine is "quantitative", traditional Chinese medicine is "qualitative". In fact, when Professor Guan elaborated more on this topic, he further said that "if a bald man only had a thin strip of hair around his ears, but this hair was good colour and 'full of lustre', then this was a sign of 'good kidneys'. Alternatively, someone who had a lot of head hair, but that hair was poor colour and lacked lustre, they undoubtedly had 'poor kidneys'".

In addition, to be sure, one must always check with the jing jing bing hou, backed with an understanding of the year, the time of the year, etc. Many misunderstood; sometimes "visual" symptoms can confuse issues.

CHAPTER 4

Winter is Bad for The Kidneys?

By now, the reader is familiar with the Chinese medicine interpretation of the term "kidneys". As for the terms "good" and "bad", the reader should also have realised the ambiguity of these terms. It is not, however, the case, as some people have formulated, that the ancient Chinese were totally amoral and didn't believe there was a "good" or "bad"; just when it came to real life and practical application, they believed extreme yin or yang were "bad" and that balance was "good".

Again, how many acupuncture and Chinese medicine students have not heard the idea that winter is bad for the kidneys? Are the modern-day Chinese doctors all wrong? No, like I've said before, they are not all wrong, but this is one of problems with "watering down" a system and taking things out of context.

Many of the original books say that the kidneys relate to winter. As far back as the *Neijing*, it was often said in these classic works that the kidneys were to cold as they were to winter. In fact, the *Qian jin fang* goes as far as saying, "In winter, the kidney water rules, its pulse is sunken soft and slippery which means balance". Furthermore, the kidneys are said to be wang (effulgent or flourishing) in winter. At best, they are "tai guo" (too much) or "bu ji" (not enough), if left alone, or perhaps "shi" (excess) or "xu" (deficient), if attacked by their respective evils; but certainly not any the worse for being involved with winter. In other words, the ancient Chinese considered winter to be a perfectly natural phenomenon.

So where does this idea of winter being bad for the kidneys come from? Essentially, what this actually relates to is the "ba feng". The "ba feng" (eight winds) are also one aspect of traditional Chinese medicine and acupuncture that revolves around the view that evil (pathogenic) wind can injure various organs and parts of the body. For example, in winter, at "dong zhi" (December 21–23 up till February 3–5 in the Northern Hemisphere), cold wind "from the North" can injure the bones, shoulders, and back (and their respective tendons).

One can imagine the implication of this, and naturally, this is where the idea of "cold is bad for the kidneys" comes from. Therefore, in conclusion, the concept that "cold is bad for the kidneys" is not as wrong as it is misunderstood and misapplied. This is an example where being generalised can lead to future problems.

CHAPTER 5

You Must Strengthen The Kidneys in the Case of Chronic Illness.

So far, we have looked at the Chinese medicine definition of the kidneys and their relationship, or lack of relationship, with baldness, cold, winter, etc. However, this time we are also asked to look at the statement "You must strengthen the kidneys in the case of chronic disease" and further ask yourselves, "Should you?"

For a long time, the present Chinese medicine hierarchy has been at great pains to "push" the notion that it is essential to strengthen or reinforce the kidneys when dealing with chronic disease. While, on the surface, this would seem a good idea, there are still many considerations we must look at. Firstly, is there such a thing as kidney "heat" or kidney "excess"? Modern Chinese medicine doctors would say "no", but we find in the *Qian jin fang* that this is far from the case. The prescriptions are listed here as follows:

<u>Xie shen tang</u>

cures kidney excess heat, small abdomen distended stuffy, four limbs black, deafness, dreams about the waist and spine li jie and hidden water, etc. qi ji prescription.

Mang xiao fu ling huang qin each 3 liang   sheng di shi chang pu each 5   liang   ci shi   8 liang dai huang 1 sheng yuan shen xi xin each 4 liang   gan cao 2 liang.

cures kidney heat very angry, very forgetful/absent-minded, ear without sounds, four limbs stuffy tense, waist back twisted and movement stiff straight prescription.

chai hu fu shen   huang qin   zhe xie sheng ma xing ren da qing   mang xiao each 2 liang ci shi 4 liang   ling yang jiao 1 liang di huang   dan zhu ye each 1 sheng

cures kidney heat, urine yellow red won't go out. When does is like cape-jasmine fruit (zhi zi) juice, or like yellow-leaf juice. Very often the urination stalk head is painful prescription.

yu bai pi dong kui zi   each 1 sheng   che qian cao 1 sheng hua shi   half sheng zi qin tong cao qu mai each 3 liang shi wei   4 liang

While most of these prescriptions are "cheng qi" and are <u>cheng qi tang</u> kinds of prescriptions, the "five elements" should tell us that if the elemental system of "sheng" (grow/create) or "ke" (destroy/counter-act) exists, then there must be kidney "heat" or kidney "excess" (see Figure 2).

Figure 2

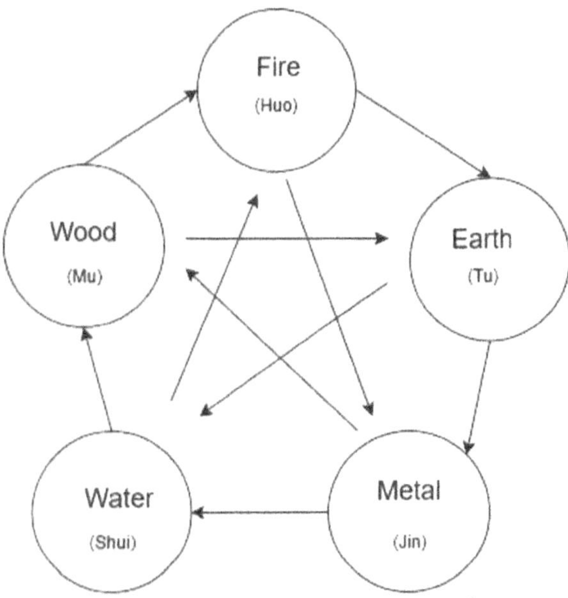

Hence, this time in closing, I will simply say that looking at the information already presented here leads me to believe that this all indicates that we are confusing one cycle with another. The Zi wu liu zhu (China Clock Therapy) chart shown in Professor Guan Zun hui's book *On the Theory and Clinical Application of Channels and Collaterals* (as featured below in Figure 3) reflects merely the ebb and flow of energy from day to day, not necessarily throughout one person's entire life.

Although kidney "heat" or kidney "excess" are problems we may encounter in the short term, the idea that "you must strengthen the kidneys in the case of chronic illness" may well be more right than wrong. Whereas, the other "proverbs" that we have looked at so far appear to be more wrong than right, depending on their particular context.

Professor Guan, when asked about a patient of mine, once asked, how old he was. Upon answering, he pointed out that because he was in his 40s when he had contracted bad cellulitis, his problem was due to kidney yin deficiency and too much phlegm due to qi stagnancy. Research, using ancient literature, appears to support this stance. The *Su wen*, for one, says, "The Tian gui (substance origins from the kidney essence necessary for regulation of growth and reproduction) of man exhausts at the age of 64 (8x8). When he is 40 (5x8), only half of his Yin energy is left over, and his actions in daily life become weak. When he is 50, his blood and energy decline and his body becomes clumsy. As the essence and blood are insufficient to nourish oneself, his eyes and ears are no more acute. At the age of 60 which is approaching 64 (8x8), his tian gui becomes exhausted, his kidney being declined and he becomes impotent. The kidney energy is the primordial true energy, when it is declined, the solid and hollow organs energies will be weakened and can no more nourish the nine orifices and they will be no more facile. Since the Yang energy below is feeble and the Yin energy above is overabundant, it causes the tears to come out. This is the case when one fails to regulate the Yin and Yang properly and causes early ageing. Therefore, when one knows how to regulate the Yin and Yang properly will make his body strong, and his body will become decrepit and senile when not knowing how to regulate it."

Furthermore, Professor Guan, in his book, reminds us that, generally, most kidney heat in the long term is due to kidney yin deficiency and fire flaring up, thereby requiring <u>huang bai</u> (Phellodendron bark) or <u>zhi mu</u> (*Anemarrhenae rhizome*) or prescriptions like <u>liu wei di huang wan,</u> etc. The classics, in addition, spend considerable time talking about nourishing the kidney yin and reducing the xiang huo (mutual fire) or, alternatively, promoting the ming men (life-gate) fire; so much so, there are two schools of thought along these lines.

Figure 3

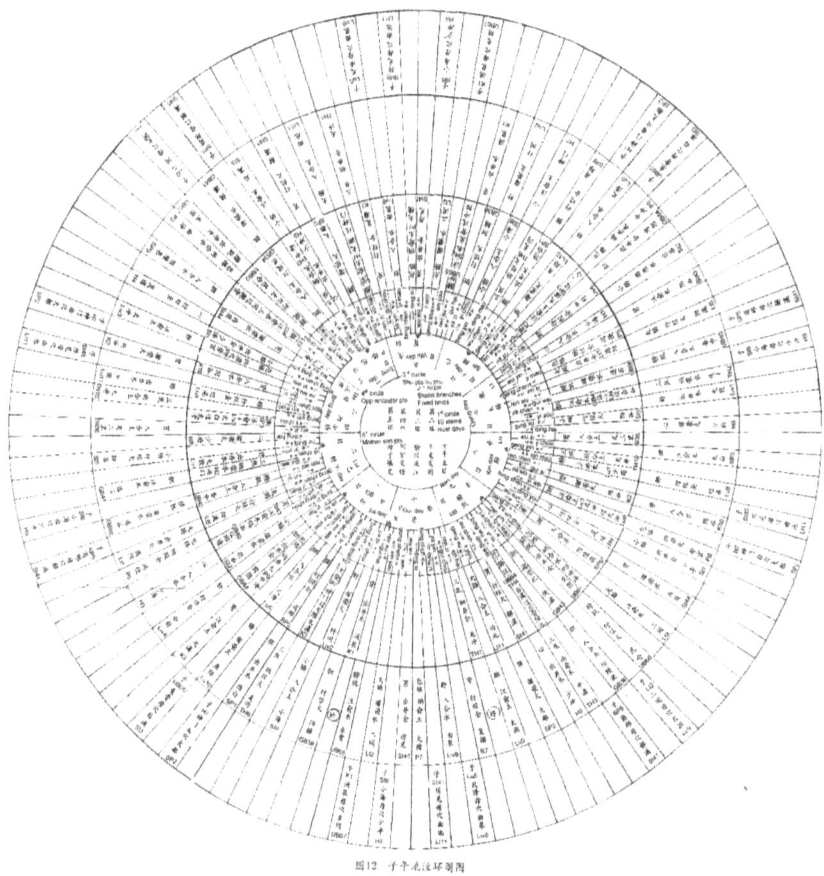

As one can see, there is a kidney "heat" and a kidney "excess", at least in the short run, which cannot be ignored, especially when dealing with years and times of years etc. However, this is one area, when *pre 1949 acupuncture* and post 1949 acupuncture tend to agree, at least in the long run. Only applications and context may really be the true points of contention.

Chapter 6

3:00–5:00 a.m. is the Time of The Lungs

So far, in the last three chapters, we have discussed a number of controversial topics. While the interpretations and conclusions of these matters may still appear somewhat ambiguous, this chapter is definitely not the case.

There are six flows of qi in the human body, as told to me by Professor Guan, and only one of these systems of qi flow is partly connected to "conscious control". This is, in fact, the qi jing ba mai (eight extraordinary channels). Its flow is not only related to "conscious control" problems but also its channels flow deep within the body and are not affected by the time of day, weather, seasons, jie qi, etc. This is the system that is extensively used in tai-chi, qi gong, etc.

On the other hand, the "saying" or adage used above (i.e., "3:00–5:00 a.m. is the time of the lungs") actually relates to another system of qi flow (see Figure 4 and Table 2). As we can see, this relates to the system of qi flow in the body called the "regular flow of qi". It starts with lungs and continues, like a cycle, within the human body, much like the mapped-out lines shown on acupuncture models and charts (see Figure 5).

Therefore, what is assumed to be very much the case is actually not. As tai-chi and qi gong is related to "conscious control" and not the "regular flow of qi", which normally flows through our bodies, this is obviously not the same. However, as I found in China, there was a Taoist monk, who was quite famous in olden times (by the name of Zhu Ge liang), who developed a system of calculating the time for doing tai chi, qi gong, ba gua, xing yi, etc. internal martial arts. Much of this system of calculating the time is quite complex, and after showing the disc (like Figure 6) to many people, I was unable to elicit any help in its use. Similar attempts, by the author, to translate it have also failed.

Yes, performing tai chi or qi gong early in the morning is quite beneficial to your health. After all, this is when the sun comes up, the animals are stirring, the cocks are crowing, and everything is indicative of "yang" rising. Alternatively, at night, everything is dark, quiet, and generally more "yin"—not a good time for any physical work or exercise. Once again (even more so), what we have now looked at shows us that the wrong understanding can be applied to the wrong situation. If we want to practice tai chi, qi gong, etc., according to time, in order to get better results, we should really know what we are doing and why.

Figure 4

The Cyclical Flow of Qi in the Twelve Regular Meridians
Exterior and interior relationships

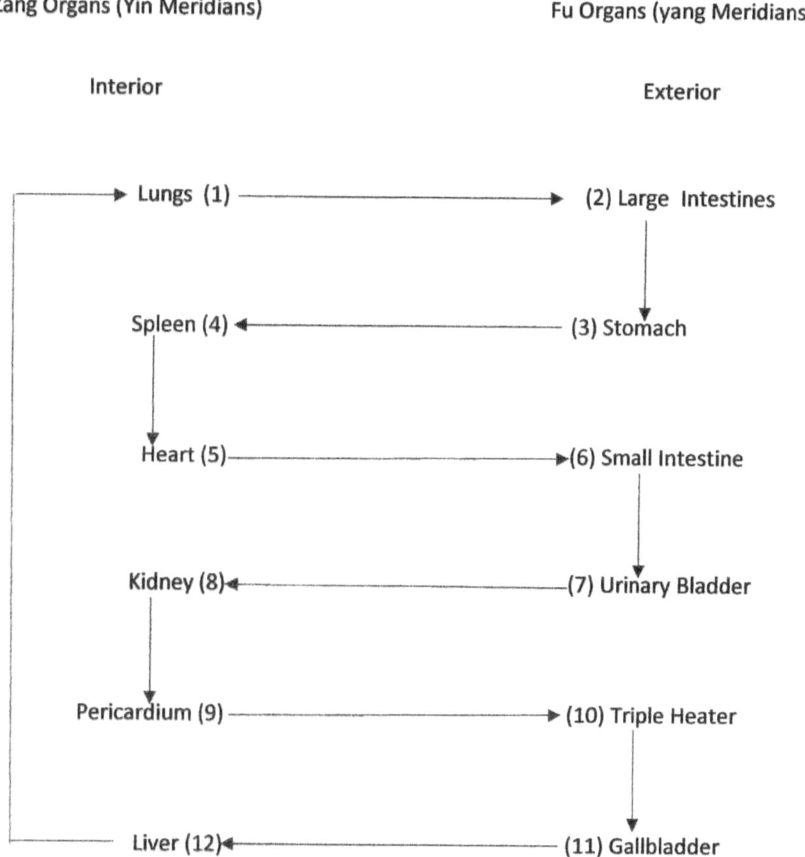

Table 2

Procedure for Tonifying the Mother Points and Sedation the Son Points:							
Meridians	Channels & the 5 Elements	What Meridian Is Active at This Time	Examples of Disease Symptoms	Law of Tonification		Law of Sedation	
				Mother Points	5 Elements Position	Mother Points	5 Elements Position
Lungs	xin metal	yin 3:00–5:00 a.m.	asthmatic cough; much phlegm; expectoration; fullness in the chest; sore throat	Lu9	earth	Lu5	water
Large Intestine	geng metal	mao 5:00–7:00 a.m.	frontal headaches; toothaches; sore throat; mouth, face, & nose diseases; upper limb paralysis	LI11	earth	LI2	water
Stomach	wu earth	chen 7:00–9:00 a.m.	distended abdomen; athlete's foot; paralysis; stomach & intestinal diseases	St 41	fire	St45	metal
Spleen	ji earth	si 9:00–11:00 a.m.	stuff tongue: greatly distended abdomen; overweight; jaundice	Sp2	fire	Sp5	metal

Heart	ding fire	wu 11:00 a.m.–1:00 p.m.	heart pain; heart palpitations; insomnia; lack of spirit or willpower; hot palms	H9	wood	H7	Earth
Small Intestines	bing fire	wei 1:00–3:00 p.m.	neck rigidity after sleeping; shoulder pain: swollen jaws; ear diseases	SI3	wood	SI8	Earth
Urinary Bladder	ren water	shen 3:00–5:00 p.m.	occipital headache; pain in neck, lumbargo region and back of knee; epilepsy	UB67	metal	UB65	Wood
Kidney	gui water	you 5:00–7:00 p.m.	lower-back pain; throat diseases; coughing up saliva with blood; little energy (qi)	k7	metal	k1	Wood
Pericardium	ding fire	xu 7:00–9:00 p.m.	spasms, cramps, or convulsions; restlessness; pain from armpits to ribs; hysterical laughter; insomnia; forgetfulness	P9	wood	P7	Earth

Triple Heater	bing fire	hai 9:00–11:00 p.m.	deathness; eye pain; throat pain; pain from armpits to ribs	TH3	wood	TH 10	Earth
Gall Bladder	jia wood	zi 11:00 p.m.–1:00 a.m.	headache on one side; ear diseases; eye pain; pain in the ribs or chest; malaria	GB43	water	GB 38	Fire
Liver	yi wood	chou 1:00–3:00 a.m.	pain in the armpit to rib region, hernia, vertical headache	Lv8	water	Lv2	Fire

Figure 5

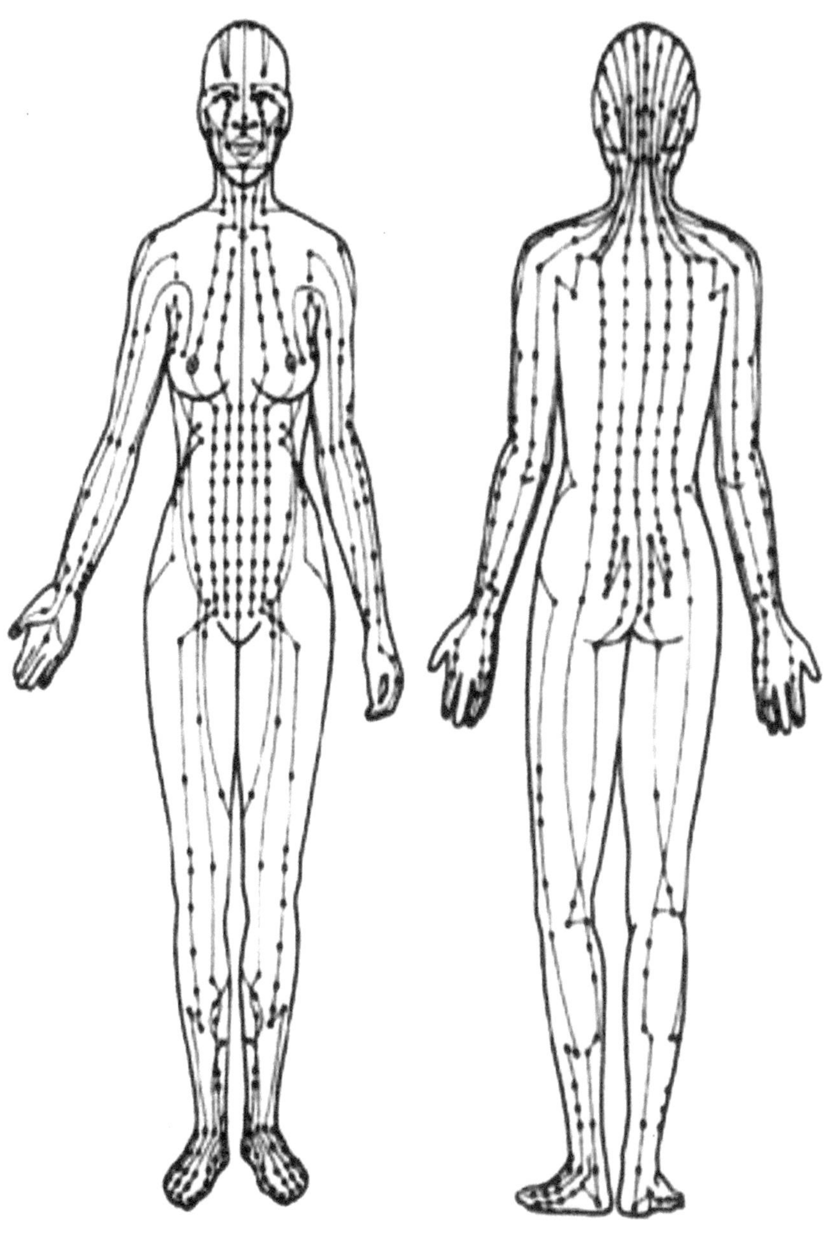

Figure 6

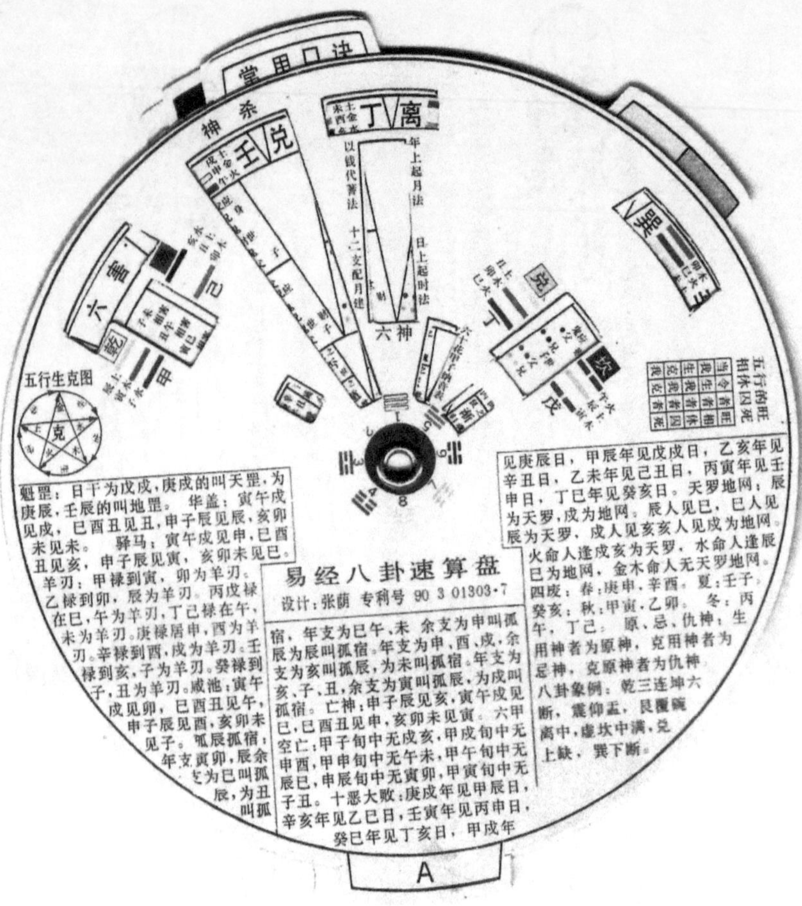

CHAPTER 7

Treatment

"Transform" and "Transport"

Obviously, some recognition must be given to emotional problems, once they have actually formed, but remember that Zhang Zhong jing considered even those problems to be the result of external factors invading and stagnating internally: i.e., wind and cold block the liver producing stagnant liver qi, stagnant liver qi transforms into fire or stagnant liver qi along with weakness of the spleen causes the production of phlegm or damage to the yuan qi results in insufficient blood (*Chinese Acupuncture and Moxibustion*, Foreign Languages Press, pp. 426–429).

This is one difference between pre and post 1949 acupuncture and Chinese medicine. (Concentrating on emotional issues is not only the providence of modern Western medicine but also treating them will fail because you are dealing with the result rather than the cause (see Figure 7).) Another difference is that recent-day acupuncture and Chinese medicine is overly concerned with "tonifying the mother" and "sedating the son.

Pre 1949 acupuncture and Chinese medicine, however, refers more to "hua" (transform) and "yun" (transport). (In some ways, though the terms are used interchangeably, "yun" can be seen as the result of "hua".) Not only is all this very different from tonifying deficiency, but it is also very different from sedating excess.

While tonifying the mother and sedating the son are part of acupuncture and Chinese medicine, regardless of pre or post 1949, it is not only just part of treating the radial pulse, but "transforming" and "transporting" also is generally considered essential for diagnosis and treating hard-to-cure disorders, especially those relating to the year and from year to year.

For example, the *Shan bu yi sheng wei lun* says, "Yuan yang stores at kan (one of the eight trigrams) residence, yun use is suitable at li (one of the eight trigrams) palace"; "Qi becomes water source, kan becomes and forms li"; "Both kidneys in between, build yang residence 2 yin's inside, therefore produces at kan".

As one can see, most of these cases of hua and yun revolve around the use of the ba gua and the eight trigrams. Professor Guan also adds, "If use 5 elements produces: beginning from zhen trigram, then the house has wood, zhen and xun produces li (fire); li (fire) produces earth (tu) kun, earth (kun) produces gold/metal (dui and qian); gold produces water (kan); water produces wood (combined with gen tu earth) . . . it demonstrates that true wood and fire produce (metal) and were born of earth . . .".

In other words, Western medicine is interested in "killing" with antibiotics; modern-day acupuncture is concerned about, almost exclusively, with tonifying and sedating; and pre 1949 acupuncture also considers hua and yun. Therefore, we not only need to remember some tonification and sedation in our treatment, but we also need to realise and understand so much more: when a situation requires actual "tonification" and "sedation", when it is simply "tai guo" (too much) or "bu ji" (not enough), when it demands some degree of hua or yun, or even a combination of the above. Our study of acupuncture is never ending. "De qi" is one such case in point.

"De qi"

"De qi" has, for a long time (at least since 1949), meant "to obtain qi" or "get qi". This is said to be achievable through one's "shou fa" (hand technique or doctor technique).

Part of the problem here is mis-translation, not just applying things "the wrong way" at the "wrong time". A better translation of "de qi" might be to "elicit" or to "enable qi".

In many ancient classics, instead of using "hua" or "yun", the "post 1949" doctors used "de". In this sense then, "de" is really the third part of the equation. While "hua" is transform and "yun" is transport, "de" is enable. In other words, "de" is closely related to hua and yun, i.e., one "gua" (trigram), or element, for that matter, can "enable" the creation of another "gua" or element.

Even this translation or interpretation, however, has problems. In truth, these things might be better called "limitations". For example, when we look at the use of CV 6 (qi hai), in the official summarisations of this point (in the book *Zhen jiu xue* wei p. 56), it tells us that if we use "de qi" in this case, it will automatically result in "sedation". In fact, in the *Tong ren shu xue zhen jiu tu jing*, it says "De qi is the same as sedation" ("de qi ji xie"). It even goes "as far" as to reiterate what Li Dong yan, etc., said that to "tonify" this point (for the purpose of increasing qi and blood), in particular, one must moxa it instead. Regardless, using "de qi" on this point and others is hardly "enabling". If one translates "de qi" as "elicit", this fits a lot better. "Eliciting qi" is one thing you wouldn't do "needling-wise", if the patient is especially weak in the first place (just as the classics state regarding the use of CV6). Therefore, we can see that "eliciting qi" is what you can or cannot do once the (yearly) qi, etc., has already properly arrived. Any attempt to draw qi to an area of the body will fail, if there is not enough qi overall. (This may be one of the reasons for "needle shock" and fainting in acupuncture practice.)

This then is the crux of the matter. Whereas, post 1949 acupuncturists talk about "de qi" as the "obtaining" or "getting" of qi, there is no way that simply needling someone will cause your qi to suddenly arrive. On the other hand, it may draw qi to the local area, but as already pointed out, this will only serve to make people weaker somewhere else. Alternatively, if a practitioner follows pre 1949 acupuncture guidelines and "elicits" qi, when the patient has enough qi to be "sourced", then it will result in a good effect. Logic would then tell us that the next step is to ensure proper arrival of qi so that we can "de qi". However, this would take longer to "go into" and is perhaps the subject of future discussion.

"Bu" and "sui", "xie" and "ying"

"De qi" are not the only words that are mis-translated, and therefore misunderstood, when looking at pre 1949 acupuncture and Chinese medicine. Bu (tonify) and xie (sedate) are also such cases. But haven't we already looked at "bu" and "xie", I hear the reader saying. While the answer is in the affirmative, I should point out that this situation is different. In the recent past, even if only a few pages ago, when we looked at "bu" and "xie", we looked at how pre 1949 acupuncture is not exclusively interested in tonifying or sedating and as interested (if not more interested) in "hua" or "yun". It was not so much mis-translation, etc.; it was more of a case of inappropriate technique selection. Here, on the other hand, we have an example of clear mis-translation and, hence, the need to re-visit these concepts again, along with "de qi".

Certainly, an understanding of "hua" and "yun" is paramount, but almost equally important too is a better understanding of "bu" and "xie". Whereas, pre 1949 acupuncture does tend to look at transformation, etc., rather than straight-out tonification and sedation, this is made all the more limited by poor translations in the past.

In modern Chinese language, "bu" means "to fill in". Furthermore, "xie" means "to drain". Ancient Chinese medicine is somewhat different: "Ying zhe, ying ze qi zhi fang sheng er duo zhi, wei xie; sui zhe, sui ze qi zhi fang xu er ji zhi. Wei bu". ("For those ying, ying its qi's position (being) flourishing and snatch, this becomes xie; for those sui, sui its qi's position xu and help (aid, relieve) it. Becomes bu".) (*Zhen jiu ci jiu fa* p. 487) This means that "xie" is the solution to "ying" (to meet, flow against), which, indeed, requires "snatching". Similarly, "xu" needs "ji" to help (or aid, relieve) one's sui (follow, come after). (In another way of putting it, "xie" is related to "duo", as is "bu" to "ji", and are both respectively involved in treating "ying" and "sui".)

The above-listed conditions are a little difficult to fully comprehend, so I have, once again, included some thoughts on the matter from Professor Guan. According to Professor Guan, you can translate "bu" as reinforce and "xie" as "reduce", as fairly commonly done these days, but it is also more pertinent that one views "bu" as "propel" and "xie" as "smoothing" the qi.

When the reader considers all the information that we have covered here, I think you will agree even "bu" and "xie", when actually called upon, are much, much more than just "tonify" and "sedate". To tonify/reinforce or to sedate/reduce not only implies that something is fixed but also relates to an absolute. Instead, we now can see how the two terms are really quite dynamic and only relate to a situation which may alternatively require "snatching" (if the moment requires it).

"Ke wo" and "wo ke"

Although we have touched upon this subject before (in *On the Theory and Practical Application of Channels and Collaterals*), I feel that no discussion of pre 1949 acupuncture would be complete without some reference to and acknowledgement of "ke wo" and "wo ke". While these areas primarily relate to the use of Zi wu liu zhu, they can, in fact, relate to other areas as well.

As the *Yi xue ren men* says, "Ke wo, wo ke ji he bi shi xue, qi xue zheng zhi shuai jue, fei qi xing wei zhi, ze qi xing ji guo, wu ci an yin xie qi, huan luan zhi qi, shi xu xu, qi huo fei xiao". ("Attack I, I attack and total bi time periods, qi and blood weakening die, qi not circling arrive, then qi circling enough too much an error needling adversely attacks evil qi, encircles a mess of true qi, excess deficiency deficiency, will cause a not so small disaster/calamity".)

Essentially, this means if the qi is weak, it will not arrive on time. Likewise, if excess (because of pathogenic factors), it will arrive too early or perhaps be chaotic. To give an example of this, should a spring pulse (i.e., Bowstring) arrive in summer (when it should be surging big), this is when a pulse (and its associated condition) has continued and failed to generate. Once more, we see pre 1949 acupuncture and Chinese medicine concerned with things arriving and not arriving on time. In other words, a critical condition or result.

In a situation of this type, the practitioner, of course, needs to resort to using Zi wu liu zhu. This is one of the things it was invented for, i.e., Qi and blood imbalances of particular types. A review of many of the classic texts shows this to be the case, and they even go so far as to say Zi wu liu zhu is one of the basic essentials or requirements of acupuncture.

Herbal medicine

While acupuncture is considered "external medicine" by the Chinese, herbal medicine is viewed as "internal medicine". In the classics, life the Nei jing, there are just as many chapters devoted to the use of herbs as there are to the practise of acupuncture. So it is little wonder that there is need to include some discussion of the subject.

As I have already said, there are many books in English which included sections on "gui jing" (channel tropism) and, additionally, systems involving the use of emperor, prime minister, and ministers. However, what many people don't know, there is also a system of combining herbs to achieve particular medicinal effects. For example, the herb jin <u>gou ji</u> (*Cibotium barometz*) and <u>chuan xu duan</u> (*Dipsacus asper*) are often used in combination to treat kidney-deficiency diarrhoea, bone problems (including breaks and contusions), and general fatigue (due to kidney jing deficiency).

Likewise, a big part of pre 1949 Chinese medicine, when treating body points, revolves around the area of taste, colour, and the nature of herbs (including when they grow long or big). There seems to be some confusion about this, particularly regarding taste. (Then again, there is also ample debate over "gui jing".) Perhaps most of this confusion is to be expected and may really stem from one thing.

This one thing is the difference between "form" and "function". Just like there are the radical pulses and their diagnosis and treatment, there are also differences between this and the treatment and diagnosis of the body points. The ancient pre 1949 Chinese medicine doctors, in other words, realised that there is the "zang" (organ) body condition, and one's zang's use (Xue gu zhen ze). At the risk of repeating myself, this is the difference between "form" and "function".

Finally, there is one part of pre 1949 Chinese herbal medicine treatment that still requires reiterating. This is, in fact, an area that we've looked at before in Professor Guan's book *On the Theory and Clinical Application of Channels and Collaterals*. Nonetheless, this is also an area of quite some significance and can't help but contribute to our complete understanding herbal medicine. While we have already looked at "gui jing" (channel tropism), herbal compatibility, taste, colour, nature (i.e., "big" or "long"), and "form" or "function", we still, however, have not looked at qi/taste "thick" or "thin". Although a more complete understanding can be obtained by referring to the above-mentioned book on this and other matters, I feel there is a more-than-adequate quote that I should mention at this point: "Qi wei you hou bo, xing yong you zao jing, zhi bao you duo shao, li hua you qian shen, ci zhi wei ye". ("The qi and taste have thick and thin, its nature have impatient and calm, treatment help have a lot and less, force transformation have shallow and deep, all so-called *Su wen-zhi zhen yao da lun*".)

All in all, and like acupuncture, Chinese herbal medicine is able to alter and affect qi and blood in the body in so many ways and on so many levels. When we get a cure, it is, therefore, not the aim. This is merely the consequence or result of balancing or treating the body.

Frequency of Treatment

Lately, I have noticed that many practitioners see patients once a week or sometimes even once a fortnight. Essentially, this is practising acupuncture commercially, not professionally. By this, I mean that a large number of practitioners, wanting to placate their patients, are mainly concerned with "metering out" expenses and charging what they think the public can afford to pay. Nothing wrong with this, I hear the reader say. True, economics and a budget are important things to consider. However, where does actually "getting people better" come into this argument? "The bottom line" is that many practitioners will swear they know what they're doing but actually don't. Hence, the need for pre 1949 acupuncture. In pre 1949 acupuncture, there is a need for "timing", along with "synchronicity". In other words, to wait a week or two between treatments, to fulfil certain treatment requirements or carry out a treatment regimen, is ludicrous, if not counterproductive.

What do I mean by this, I further hear the reader ask. When asking Professor Guan about "frequency" of treatment, he reported that, in China, they have done a lot of research into the matter which shows that a patient's condition improve after receiving an acupuncture treatment, but after two to three days, this starts to subside. To counteract this and to enable the patient to get better more completely, another acupuncture treatment is needed soon after.

In order to reach some sort of satisfactory conclusion, which at the same time will promote a more "professional" outcome, I propose practitioners treat patients, particularly chronic ones, two to three times per week and then opt for a break after a three-week period for approximately two weeks. It should be possible, from this, for the patient and the practitioner to see if there are any improvements at the end of this process and whether future or fairly immediate courses of treatment are warranted.

In some cases, however, this is not always going to be the case. Very acute cases (like acute lumbago, ankle sprain, and torticollis), for example, may require treatment every day or even more frequently. Once, I had a patient with Parkinson's disease who ultimately needed five treatments a week. After four weeks of treatment, he reported that he was able to control his arm and hand-shaking with his own brain.

The only things to still discuss then, in closing, are other factors which may have a bearing on treatments and their frequency. When observing patients being treated in China, Professor Guan would often combine not only different forms of acupuncture but also different therapies. By this, I mean to say that not simply would he combine ear acupuncture (using vacarria seeds) with body acupuncture, bee acupuncture (if proven non-allergic) with Zu wu liu zhu (China clock therapy) for treating non-heat type rheumatoid arthritis, scalp acupuncture with body acupuncture for treating apoplexy, and also body points with suture acupuncture or point-injection therapy for treating a variety of chronic problems, but that he would additionally use body acupuncture combined with physiotherapy or body acupuncture combined with massage (an mo). This, in turn, would have to affect the frequency of treatments. People partaking in this level of therapy would have to have less treatments. Then again, to avoid the need for, as well as the ill effects, of surgery, one may need these fairly frequently anyway.

CHAPTER 8

The Rope

I have decided at this point in the book to do something fairly unprecedented. Usually, a final chapter on treatment would be and should be all that an author of a Chinese medicine book is required to provide. However, in this case, I have also decided to include this chapter, which I have entitled "The Rope".

As well as helping with "diagnosing" (i.e., in the sense that we need to know how to look at human beings and get some true perspective), the practitioner may also need assistance with "treatment"; not the actual act of "treatment", which we looked at last chapter, instead, again, a discussion about "perspective" when it comes to our overall approach to disease treatment. What are we really seeking to achieve when we see someone? In other words, what is the "door" behind the "door"?

To this end, I have chosen an analogy from some of the olden books of Chinese medicine. Many pre 1949 doctors believe that when we are confronted by very difficult and chronic cases, we are viewing something not all far removed from a "rope" or "sash". This "rope" or "sash", suspended from the ceiling, is not just "thick" and "strong" in some parts but also "thin", "weak", and "frail" in other parts. Likewise, doctors of Chinese medicine are often confronted by cases which are seemingly contradictory and "at loggerheads with each other". Admittedly, yin and yang are already like this in the first place. However, even the "complimentary-opposite" nature surrounding the meanings of these two terms does not explain the complex problems that people seem to have these days. For example, it is possible for people to have an excess condition with some channels and organs while, at the same time, have deficiency in other channels and organs. Furthermore, it is possible for one channel alone to suffer excesses and deficiencies at the same time. How is this possible, you ask. Professor Guan, in answer, tells us that sometimes you must sedate parts of, say, the kidney channel, and sometimes you must tonify other parts of the same channel.

So parts of the body need to be strengthened and parts need to be sedated. And then there are those which need to be sedated first and tonified later (like the "yang within yin"), and there are also those which need to be tonified first and sedated later (like often, in the cases of "yin within yang"). The number of permutations can be endless, as can be the "twists", "thicknesses", and "slenderness" of a rope (see Figure 7). Our ultimate aim, you see, is to make this "rope" or "sash" not too thick and not too thin. If we have a homogeneous "rope", we have a "balanced" patient in all senses of the word.

Figure 7

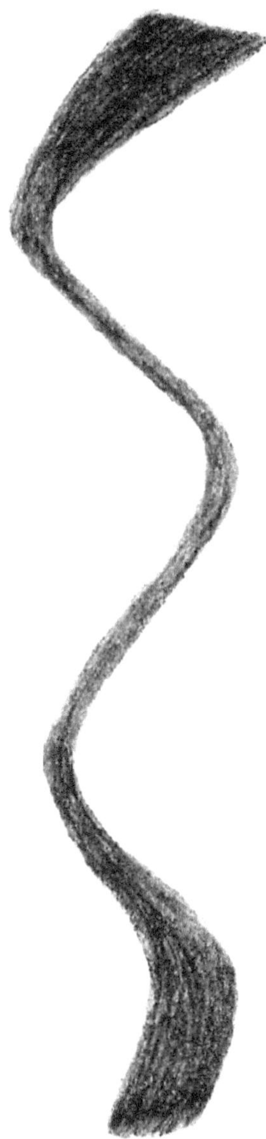

LIST OF TERMS

Ni – adverse, inverse, perverse. Both "deficient" and "excess".

Wang – flare-up. Similar to "ni" but generally more excessive, overly hot or flourishing in nature.

Wang – another character and another type of "wang", meaning "Emperor", i.e., In the winter, the kidneys are wang.

De – e.g., De qi. Enable elicit, activate.

Hua – transform. One element can transform into another.

Yun – transport. Very similar to "hua" and goes hand in hand with it. In some ways, considered the result of hua.

Ying – counter-sequential. "Ying" implies "to flow against".

Duo – to "snatch".

Sui – sequential, i.e., "to flow with".

Ji – to assist, help, aid.

Ke wo – "kill I".

Wo Ke – "I kill".

Gui ging – channel tropism.

Qi thick – governs floating, e.g., <u>fu zi</u>, <u>gan jiang</u>, <u>rou gui</u>.

Qi thin – governs raising, e.g., <u>ma huang</u>, <u>chai hu</u>, <u>sheng ma</u>, <u>ge gen</u>.

Taste thick – governs sinking, e.g., <u>dai huang</u>, <u>mang xiao</u>, <u>huang lian</u>, <u>huang bai</u>.

Taste thin – governs downwards, e.g., <u>fu ling</u>, <u>tong cao</u>, <u>zhe xie</u>, <u>chuan shan jia</u>, <u>shi jueming</u>.

RECOMMENDED READING

Huang di Nei jing

Jin Qian fang by Sun Si miao

On the Theory and Clinical Application of Channels and Collaterals by Guan Zun hui

Pi wei lun by Li Dong yan

Shan bu yi sheng wei lun by Li Zhong zi

Shang Han lun by Zhang Zhong jing

Tong ren shu xue zhen ji tu jing by Wang Wei yi

Wai tai Mi yao fang by Wang Tao

Xue gu zhen ze, 1991

Yi jing

Zhen jiu ci jiu fa, 2004

Zhen jiu jia yi jing by Huang Fu mi

Zhong guo yi xue zhen fa da jin, 1991

Zhu bing yuan hou lun

ANDREW MCPHERSON

Andrew McPherson has a BA (Modern Asian Studies) degree from Griffith University and is a government-recognised member of AHPRA. He has been a doctor of Chinese medicine for some 30 years or more. He is the president of ANACHA (Australian National Acupuncturists and Chinese Herbalists Association) and has written numerous articles for newspapers, magazines, and books. In addition, he has studied in the People's Republic of China for extended periods and is a long-term student of Professor Guan Zun hui.